MW01108257

The Library of Sexual Health™

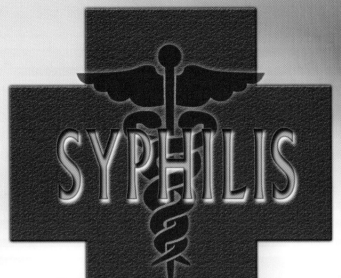

SYPHILIS

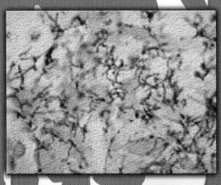

ADAM WINTERS

The Rosen Publishing Group, Inc., New York

To A. Airão: pela paciência

Published in 2007 by The Rosen Publishing Group, Inc.
29 East 21st Street, New York, NY 10010

First Edition

Library of Congress Cataloging-in-Publication Data

Winters, Adam, 1966–
Syphilis/Adam Winters.
    p. cm.—(The library of sexual health)
Includes index.
ISBN-13: 978-1-4042-0906-0
ISBN-10: 1-4042-0906-9 (library binding)
1. Syphilis—Juvenile literature. I. Title. II. Series.
RC201.W76 2006
616.95'13—dc22

                                                  2006004015

Manufactured in the United States of America

CONTENTS

Introduction 4

Chapter One | What Is Syphilis? 7

Chapter Two | Origins of Syphilis 14

Chapter Three | Diagnosing Syphilis 22

Chapter Four | Treating Syphilis 32

Chapter Five | Complications 39

Chapter Six | Prevention 46

Glossary 56

For More Information 57

For Further Reading 60

Bibliography 61

Index 63

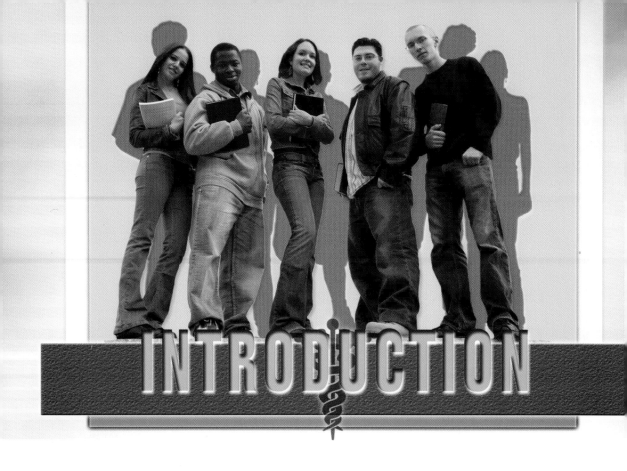

INTRODUCTION

Most young people have heard about sexually transmitted diseases (STDs) and know that STDs come from having sex with an infected person without using proper protection, such as a latex condom. Despite this knowledge, every year in North America, approximately one in four sexually active teenagers gets an STD. In the United States alone, this means that around three million teens are infected each year.

One of these STDs is syphilis. Over the centuries, the horrible consequences of untreated syphilis in its later stages made it a feared disease. Society often viewed those who suffered from it as sinful or shameful. Today, syphilis

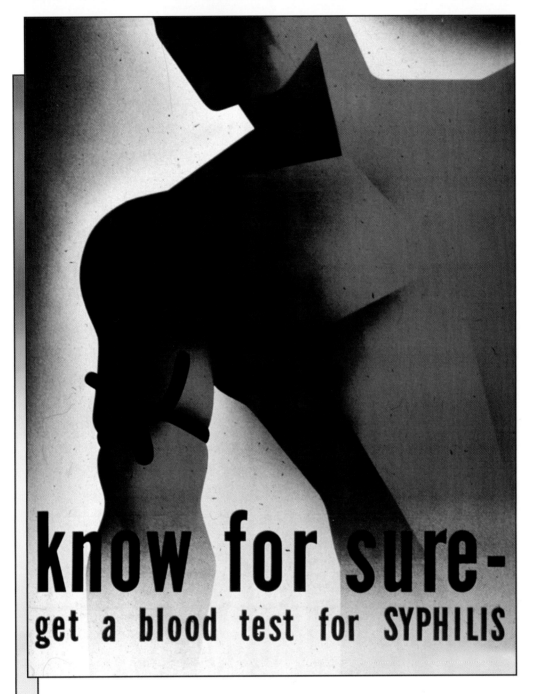

know for sure -
get a blood test for SYPHILIS

This poster was printed and distributed by the U.S. Public Health Service during World War II. At the time, syphilis was significantly more common than it is today, and there was no effective treatment.

is still feared. However, while many young people have heard of this infection, few know much about it.

A major reason for this lack of information is that in recent years syphilis infections had become quite rare in North America. In fact, in the late 1990s, medical experts and health officials in Canada and the United States foresaw a twenty-first century in which syphilis would be eliminated altogether. In the last few years, however, both countries have seen a new rise in cases of syphilis. Most of those infected have been young people, who lack knowledge about the disease and how it is transmitted. This is unfortunate, because awareness is key when dealing with a disease whose signs are often very hard to detect. The truth is that many people acquire syphilis without even knowing it. On the positive side, tests for syphilis are quick and efficient. If detected early, the disease is easy to treat and leaves no lasting effects.

This book aims to provide solid information that will help young people avoid acquiring and transmitting syphilis, while informing those who are already infected— or think they might be—about how to get diagnosed and cured. Hopefully, armed with this knowledge, we will be one step closer to wiping out syphilis for good.

CHAPTER ONE

What Is Syphilis?

Syphilis is a serious but curable infection caused by bacteria called *Treponema pallidum*. Bacteria are simple microscopic organisms that are the oldest form of life on Earth. They are highly adaptable and can live anywhere—at the bottom of the ocean, in frigid Arctic ice, and in steamy hot springs, as well as in any kind of plant or animal species. The wormlike bacterium that causes syphilis, for example, likes to burrow into the moist mucous membranes of human beings' mouths or genital areas.

You can get syphilis by coming into contact with a person who already has the disease. Most of the time, this occurs as a result of sexual activity, which is why syphilis is considered an STD. Syphilis can be transmitted either through oral, genital, or anal sex. Even partners who don't engage in actual sexual penetration—of a penis into a vagina, for example—can still get syphilis.

Syphilis is spread when one person's infected area, usually an open sore, touches the soft skin of the mucous membrane found inside or around another person's genital or anal areas, or in or around the mouth. A mucous membrane is a special protective layer of skin that safeguards the body's internal passages and certain cavities from the outside environment. It lines the skin of nostrils, lips, ears, genitals, and the anus, and helps the body to absorb and secrete fluids. When stimulated, these membranes give off

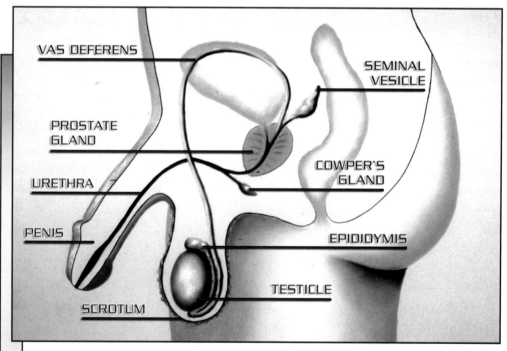

This profile view of a male body shows the reproductive organs. These organs—the penis, scrotum, urethra, testicle, vas deferens, prostate gland, seminal vesicle, epididymis, and Cowper's gland—work together to produce and release semen during sexual intercourse. The male reproductive system also produces sex hormones, which help a boy develop into a sexually mature man.

a sticky, thick fluid called mucus (such as what comes out of our noses when we sneeze) that moistens and protects.

Although less common, syphilis can also be spread through needle sharing (which occurs among drug users) and by an infected person coming into contact with any type of open sore or cut on another person. A pregnant woman with syphilis can also infect the unborn baby

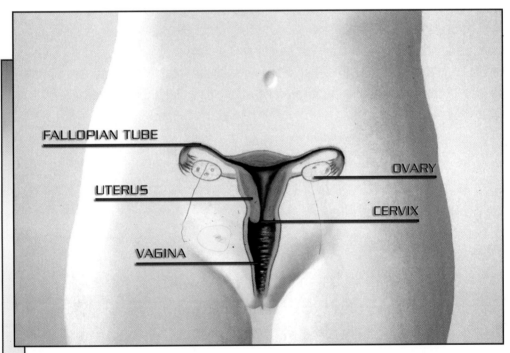

This illustration shows the female reproductive organs. From top to bottom are the fallopian tubes, ovaries, uterus, cervix, and vagina. The female reproductive system allows a woman to have sexual intercourse, produce eggs, and protect and nourish a fertilized egg until it becomes a baby.

MYTH: If you use a condom, you can't get syphilis.
FACT: Syphilis can be transmitted to and from areas that are not covered or protected by a latex condom.

MYTH: Once you've had syphilis and been treated for it, you can never get it again.
FACT: You can be infected with syphilis a second time (or more) if an exposed area or open wound comes into contact with someone else's infection.

MYTH: Syphilis can be spread through contact with doorknobs, toilet seats, swimming pools, and bathtubs, or by sharing clothing or eating utensils.
FACT: Syphilis can be transmitted only when an open sore comes into direct contact with an area of broken skin or mucous membranes where body fluids are exposed.

she is carrying. Syphilis acquired in this manner is known as congenital syphilis.

TREPONEMES

There are actually several forms of syphilis. The most serious is the sexually transmitted variety discussed in this book, caused by *Treponema pallidum*. This spiral-shaped bacterium is one of a related group of bacteria known as the treponemes.

Other treponemes cause milder infections that aren't sexually transmittable. These are usually skin infections that often affect young children. Scientists believe that sexually transmittable syphilis probably evolved from one of these other forms, though precisely when this might have occurred remains a mystery.

RECENT OUTBREAKS

Until recently, outbreaks of syphilis were fairly rare, especially in North America. However, in the last decade,

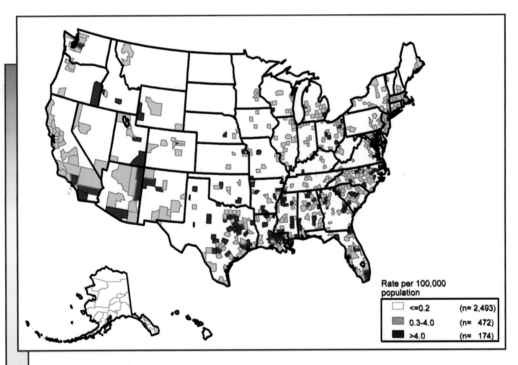

Rate per 100,000 population

☐ <=0.2	(n= 2,493)
▨ 0.3-4.0	(n= 472)
■ >4.0	(n= 174)

Since 2000, cases of syphilis have been steadily rising, particularly in North American cities and among men of all ethnic groups. In 2004, for the third year in a row, San Francisco had the highest syphilis rate of any U.S. city. The map above shows American cities where rates of primary and secondary (P&S) stages of syphilis are the highest.

"The Lost Children" — A Case Study

In 1999, the PBS television program *Frontline* aired a documentary titled "The Lost Children of Rockdale County." The film focused on a 1996 syphilis outbreak among teenagers living in a well-off suburb of Atlanta, Georgia. Through interviews with health officials, doctors, teachers, parents, and the teenagers themselves, the filmmakers explored how more than 200 adolescents—some as young as twelve years old—were exposed to the STD and the impact it had on everyone's lives. What shocked many of the health officials who investigated the outbreak was that what happened with Rockdale's teens was also occurring elsewhere in North America.

The film offered a disturbing portrait of teenage sexual behavior. At the center of the syphilis outbreak was a group of young girls who were mainly under sixteen. Most came from stable homes and excelled in school. However, many felt bored and were eager to prove themselves, both to their friends and to boys, by engaging in sexual activities. From time to time, the girls would invite groups of older boys (usually between seventeen and twenty-one) to their homes when no parents were around. After drinking alcohol and using drugs, they would spend several hours engaging in sexual activities. This was generally done in front of one another, with both girls and boys having various partners. Most of the teens' parents never suspected anything. In fact, this behavior was only discovered once infected teens began seeking medical attention and local health officials became alarmed at the astounding rate of young people infected with syphilis.

In interviews, Rockdale County's teens talked openly about their experiences and feelings. They claimed that they were never forced to have sex, but they did feel pressure—from their friends and themselves—to engage in sex in order to feel as if they belonged and to prove that they were mature. Although some teens were curious and eager to have sex for the first time, they were disappointed by the experience. After having had sex once, many felt they couldn't say no to second, third, or more times, even though, after a while, most were no longer enjoying themselves. None of the sex was accompanied by love or romantic feelings. Aside from catching and spreading a dangerous disease, a number of the teens, especially the girls, ended up feeling alone and unsatisfied. They wondered if these sexual experiences were going to affect the rest of their lives.

health officials have been concerned by statistics showing an increase in the number of syphilis cases.

According to the Public Health Agency of Canada, between 1997 and 2002, the number of syphilis cases in Canada quadrupled. And since 2003, it has continued to rise. Meanwhile, the American Centers for Disease Control and Prevention (CDC) states that in 2002, the United States registered over 32,000 cases of syphilis, a 12.4 percent increase from 2001. The highest rate of people infected were from the most sexually active group (between twenty and thirty-nine years old). In both countries, men tend to get syphilis at higher rates than women, but the women who are infected are usually younger (in the United States, syphilis is highest in females between the ages of twenty and twenty-four).

These findings are troubling. They reveal that, despite greater access to and knowledge about safer sex methods such as condoms, an increasing number of people are having unprotected sex.

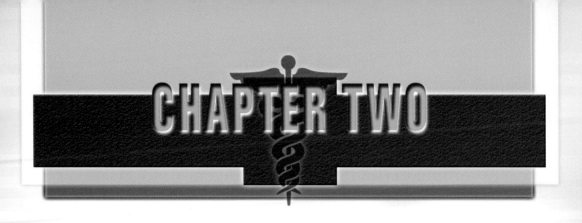

CHAPTER TWO

Origins of Syphilis

S yphilis has existed for thousands of years. The oldest traces of the disease were found in the bones of a bear that lived 11,000 years ago in what is today the state of Indiana. Meanwhile, skeletal remains found in present-day Colorado date back some 2,000 years and are the oldest known evidence of syphilis in human beings.

New World Versus Old World

More difficult for scientists to agree upon is where syphilis came from. At one time, most experts believed that it originated in the Americas and was brought to Europe by the explorer Christopher Columbus and his crew. In 1493, Columbus and his crew spent time on the island of Hispaniola (today divided between Haiti and the Dominican Republic). While there, they engaged in sexual activity with local women who were likely infected with syphilis. Researchers have discovered ample evidence dating back from 1,200 to 500 years ago of syphilis in human skeletons from this Caribbean region.

However, recent findings have challenged the view that syphilis originated in the New World. Archaeologists have uncovered ancient skeletons in Israel as well as England, Italy, and other parts of Europe whose remains show signs of syphilis, such as swollen leg bones and damaged skulls. The skeletons clearly predate Columbus's voyage and would seem to prove that syphilis existed for centuries on both sides of the Atlantic.

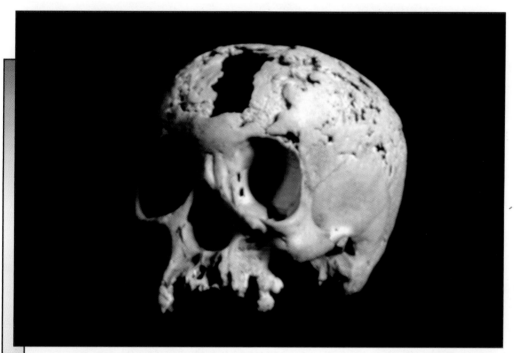

In the eighteenth and nineteenth centuries, Europe experienced a population explosion that resulted in overcrowding and poor hygiene, especially in larger cities. As a consequence, syphilis cases increased enormously. The skull of a young Englishwoman (above) who lived during the 1700s shows the destruction caused by untreated syphilis. The skull's moth-eaten appearance was caused by syphilitic lesions that ate away at the jaw and nasal bones.

Historians agree that it was following Columbus's return to Europe that syphilis began to spread at alarming rates throughout the Old World. The first recorded major outbreak of syphilis took place in the kingdom of Naples (part of today's Italy) in the 1490s. From there, it quickly swept across Europe, infecting and killing a vast number of victims.

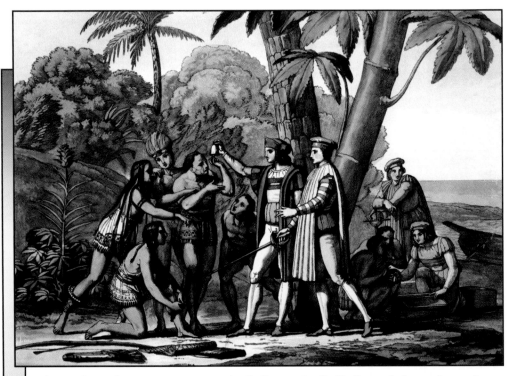

This eighteenth-century engraving by Italian artist D. K. Bonatti shows the explorer Christopher Columbus and his Spanish crew arriving in the New World. Between 1492 and 1504, Columbus made four voyages across the Atlantic, including three to the island of Hispaniola.

A Disease of Many Names

Over the years, syphilis has acquired many names and nicknames. When it first began spreading through Europe in the sixteenth century, it was called "the Great Pox." This name distinguished it from another serious disease of the time, smallpox (early symptoms of both infections included similar skin rashes). When King Charles VIII of France invaded Naples in 1495, the Neapolitans (residents of Naples) blamed the French soldiers for transmitting syphilis, which subsequently became known as "the French disease." In retaliation, the French referred to it as the "Neapolitan (or Italian) disease." Citizens of other nations also blamed the spread of syphilis on their enemies. As such, many Russians called it "the Polish disease," while Arabs called it "the disease of the Christians." And since some blamed Columbus and his crew for having brought the mysterious illness from the New World, syphilis was also commonly known as "the Spanish disease."

National conflicts aside, for a long time syphilis was known as "lues" (pronounced like the name Louise). In more recent times, it has earned nicknames ranging from "bad blood" and "syph" to "Miss Siff."

A SINFUL CONDITION

The name "syphilis" was coined by a poet and astronomer named Girolamo Fracastoro (1478–1553), who lived in the city of Verona in northern Italy. Although Fracastoro was also one of the leading physicians of his time, originally he had no idea what caused syphilis or how it was transmitted. So he decided to invent a myth that explained the origins of the disease. He did this in the form of an elegant and very long poem (it contained 1,300 verses) that he

Ten Facts About Syphilis

1. Syphilis has been around for thousands of years.

2. Syphilis is on the rise again after having almost disappeared.

3. Most new cases of syphilis are contracted by people under the age of thirty.

4. One in four sexually active teens is infected with an STD every year in North America.

5. Men tend to get syphilis at higher rates than women (up to three males for every female).

6. Most people spread syphilis to others without even knowing they have the disease.

7. If detected early, syphilis is easy to treat and leaves no lasting effects.

8. Since the 1940s, the antibiotic penicillin has been the only efficient cure for syphilis.

9. Between 40 and 70 percent of babies whose mothers have syphilis contract the disease.

10. People with syphilis are up to five times more likely to contract HIV, the virus that causes AIDS.

wrote in Latin. The poem's title was *Syphilis, sive morbus Gallicus*, which in English translates to "Syphilis, or the French Disease." (Since Verona was Naples's ally, Fracastoro was quite anti-French in his sentiments.)

The main character of the poem was a king's shepherd named Syphilus, who lived in a fictional kingdom in the New World. When Apollo, the sun god, caused a great heat wave to dry up the king's land and pastures, Syphilus was

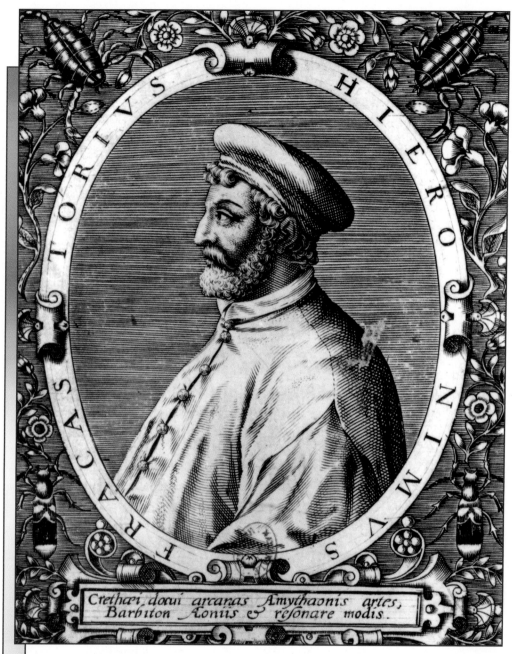

TORIVS HIERO NIMVS FRACAS

Crethæi docui arcanas Amythaonis artes,
Barbiton Aoniis & resonare modis.

This sixteenth-century engraving shows a portrait of Girolamo Fracastoro, the first person to suggest that invisible germs spread disease. Fracastoro's advanced medical discoveries helped make unpopular public health practices, such as cleaning or burning a sick person's infected clothing and bedding, more acceptable in European society.

enraged. Loyal to his king, the shepherd cursed Apollo and destroyed the altars where the god was worshiped. Apollo was so infuriated by the shepherd's actions that he decided to inflict a terrible disease on all the king's people, but first and foremost upon Syphilus. And it is hence that the name of Fracastoro's fictional shepherd became the name of one of the world's best-known illnesses (although the English spelling was changed to "syphilis").

At the time that he wrote this poem, Fracastoro, like many physicians of the day, believed that syphilis and other diseases were spread from one person to another via contagious particles carried by currents of "bad" air. However, in the years following the poem's 1530 publication, Fracastoro continued to study syphilis. He discovered that the syphilis infection takes place "only when two bodies join in most intense mutual contact, as primarily occurs in coitus [sex]." He also recognized that mothers with syphilis could pass the disease to their children, at birth or during breast-feeding. His breakthrough discovery was included in his influential scientific text *On Contagion and Contagious Diseases and Their Cure*, which was published in 1546.

Although in Fracastoro's poem the disease is seen as divine punishment for human misbehavior, Fracastoro himself did not accept this view. During the early 1500s, however, and even in the centuries that followed, many people did believe that syphilis was God's way of punishing sinners. Once it became known that the source of the disease was sexual activity (in many cases probably outside of marriage, an act that the Christian Church considered a serious sin), this view of syphilis only increased. People who acquired syphilis were treated like social outcasts. If they got very sick, or even died, it was believed to be a fate they deserved.

Unfortunately, to a certain degree, such attitudes still remain. Even today, many people who contract the disease are often made to feel sinful and guilty by society at large. Sadly, such fears of being judged drive many people, particularly teens, to avoid getting diagnosed and treated for syphilis. It also results in them spreading the disease to other unsuspecting partners, either because they are ashamed to get tested or afraid of confessing to others that they are, or might be, infected.

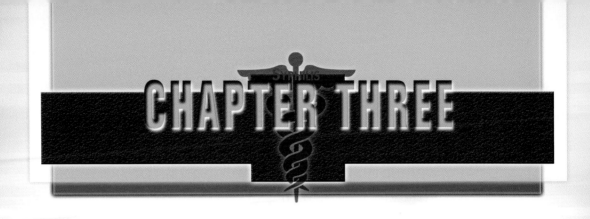

CHAPTER THREE

Diagnosing Syphilis

Syphilis is sometimes referred to as the "great imitator." This is because the disease has numerous symptoms (physical signs that allow doctors to positively diagnose or identify an infection) that can often be confused with those of other illnesses. Since until recently cases of syphilis in North America were uncommon, doctors sometimes overlooked it as a possible diagnosis.

STAGES AND SYMPTOMS

If left untreated, syphilis moves through various phases, each characterized by specific symptoms. Most medical experts usually identify syphilis as having four separate stages: primary, secondary, latent, and tertiary.

Primary Syphilis

During the primary, or first, stage of syphilis, the classic sign of the disease is a painless open sore. Called a chancre (rhymes with "anchor"), this sore will appear at the site where the syphilis bacteria entered the body. Since infection usually occurs as a result of sexual contact, the chancre will appear around the genital area, anus, lips, mouth, or throat. It is frequently firm, round, small, and hard-edged. Sometimes, several chancres might appear.

Chancres can emerge anytime between ten days and three months following infection. On average, they form around three weeks after the syphilis enters your body. The sore is painless, so you probably won't feel it. If you

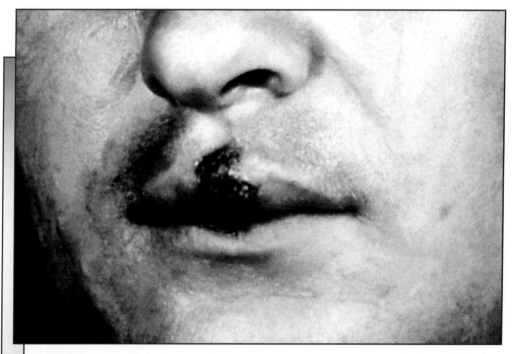

A lip chancre *(above)* is a typical symptom of syphilis in its primary stage. Chancres appear at the spot where syphilis entered the body and last about three to six weeks.

or somebody else doesn't see it (if it's hidden around your genital area, for example), you might never know you're infected. In fact, this is frequently the case, which is why it is important to be tested regularly for syphilis. The sore, which usually lasts between three and six weeks, will often go away on its own without treatment. However, the infection will remain inside your body. During this stage the bacteria are infectious, meaning that you can pass the disease on to someone else through sexual contact. Most people transmit syphilis to others without even knowing they have it.

Secondary Syphilis

If syphilis is not detected and treated during the primary stage, there is around a 30 percent chance that it will progress to the secondary stage. The signs of secondary syphilis can appear while the first-stage chancre is still healing, or weeks later. The symptoms of secondary syphilis are more serious and also more varied. They can include any of the following: fever; patchy hair loss; aching muscles and joints; swollen glands; sore throat; headaches; weight loss; lack of energy; rashes on the soles of the feet, the palms of the hands, or elsewhere on the body; and lesions (wounds) on mucous membranes.

Usually, the most common symptoms of secondary syphilis, and the first to appear, are the skin rashes and lesions. Rashes might break out on various parts of the body, but more often than not, they don't itch. Typically, rashes on the soles of the feet and palms of the hands are rough in texture and red or reddish brown in color. However, on other parts of the body, they often resemble those that accompany many other conditions. Sometimes the rashes are so faint that they are near impossible to detect. If left untreated, these symptoms, like those for primary syphilis, will usually disappear on their own.

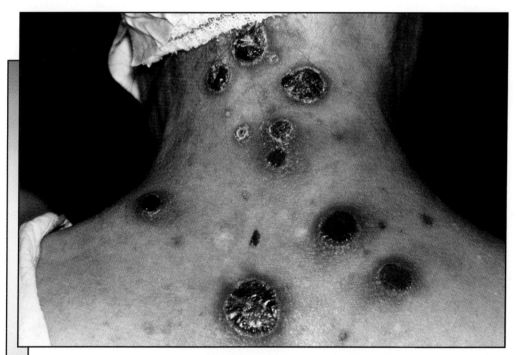

The rash on this patient's back and neck is one of the most common symptoms of syphilis in its secondary stage. Rashes can be either flat or raised, and usually do not hurt or itch. During secondary syphilis, the *Treponema pallidum* bacteria may multiply until more than 500 million are spread throughout the body.

Regardless of what symptoms you have, secondary syphilis is the stage where the syphilis bacteria have spread throughout the bloodstream and have reached their highest numbers. This means that the second stage is the most contagious, and your chances of passing the disease to somebody else are highest.

Latent Stage

The latent stage of syphilis begins when the second-stage symptoms disappear. An illness is latent when its symptoms are hidden or invisible. However, the infection still remains in the body. This is the case with syphilis if it is not treated during the first or second stages. It can remain latent in the body for months and often years. In many cases, it will simply remain inactive. Unless you get tested for syphilis, you'll never even know you have the disease. Although during the first twelve months or so of latent syphilis you can still infect other people, after around a year the disease stops being contagious.

Tertiary Stage

The tertiary, or third, stage of syphilis is the final and most feared phase of the disease. In around 25 percent of people with latent syphilis, the active bacteria will eventually begin to do serious damage to internal organs, including the brain, heart, nerves, eyes, liver, bones, joints, and blood vessels. Often, this damage won't be detected for a long time. It might take years to show up. When symptoms of tertiary syphilis do finally emerge, however, they can be very serious and frightening. These symptoms include difficulty coordinating muscle movements, numbness, paralysis, gradual blindness, and dementia (insanity).

While syphilis itself can still be treated at this stage, these symptoms are so serious that the damage they inflict can't always be repaired. Often, internal organs such as

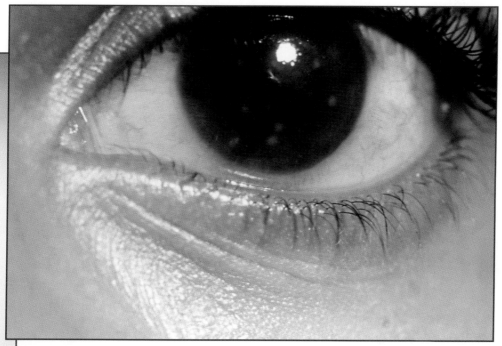

The white spots in this person's eye show interstitial corneal keratitis, a serious eye condition that is a common symptom of later stages of acquired and congenital syphilis. If not treated, this condition, which is the leading cause of blindness in the world, can result in serious sight problems and a total loss of vision.

Famous Syphilis Cases

Since the symptoms of syphilis are common to many diseases, it is difficult to know for sure if certain key historic figures were infected with the disease. Aside from Christopher Columbus, however, famous personalities that some historians believe suffered from syphilis include composers Franz Schubert and Wolfgang Amadeus Mozart; poet Charles-Pierre Baudelaire; novelists Gustave Flaubert, Leo Tolstoy, and Fyodor Dostoyevsky; painters Édouard Manet and Paul Gauguin; Chicago gangster Al Capone; and world leaders ranging from the French emperor Napoléon and Russia's King Ivan "the Terrible" to U.S. president Woodrow Wilson and Nazi dictator Adolf Hitler.

the liver, heart, and brain can suffer great harm. In fact, if allowed to reach an advanced stage, tertiary syphilis can lead to death.

TESTING FOR SYPHILIS

It is often difficult to diagnose syphilis based solely on symptoms of the first two stages. In the end, the most reliable way of finding out about infection is to get tested at a clinic or by your doctor. If you even remotely suspect that you might have syphilis, the last thing you should feel is afraid. You should never feel ashamed or embarrassed about getting tested for syphilis. If you don't have the disease, you will feel great relief. If you do, you will save both yourself and future partners from potential physical discomfort and harm as well as considerable emotional stress.

If you think you have syphilis, talk to your parents or another adult you trust, such as your family doctor or the school nurse. You can also call your local public health department or Planned Parenthood clinic and ask about testing. In many states, you can go to a health clinic and have a syphilis test done without your parents' consent. If you are worried about this, call the clinic beforehand. Ask

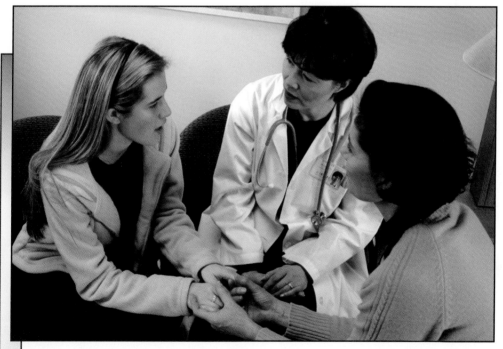

Here, a doctor explains a syphilis diagnosis to a teenager and her mother. Although health workers are skilled at dealing with young patients who are diagnosed with STDs, it can help to bring a friend or family member with you for emotional support.

Ten Great Questions to Ask Your Doctor
After You've Been Diagnosed with Syphilis

1. How can I have syphilis if I didn't notice any symptoms?

2. Is there a cure for syphilis, or will I always have the disease?

3. Do I need to be tested for HIV and other STDs?

4. Can I currently infect other people even if I have no symptoms?

5. Do I have to tell sexual partners (present and past) that I have syphilis?

6. Should I urge them to get tested as well?

7. Can I engage in sexual activity while I'm being treated?

8. Will treatment make all of my symptoms go away?

9. If my symptoms disappear, does that mean that the syphilis is gone?

10. After I've been treated for syphilis, does that mean I can never get it again?

if you need to bring your parent along for permission and what information the clinic will share with them.

The easiest and most common way of detecting syphilis is from a blood test. Blood tests are safe, highly accurate, and inexpensive. Shortly after becoming infected, the body naturally begins to produce syphilis antibodies in order to fight the foreign bacteria causing the infection. A low level of antibodies will stay in the blood for months and sometimes years, even after the disease has been successfully treated. Traces of these antibodies in the bloodstream will show up in any blood test, revealing whether syphilis is present or not.

Another way of testing for syphilis is by taking a sample from a possible syphilis chancre. By examining it under a microscope, a doctor can see whether syphilis bacteria are present.

Try not to feel nervous about getting tested. Remember that nurses and doctors perform such tests all the time. They are not there to judge you, but to help you. In the event that either test reveals the presence of syphilis, you shouldn't feel afraid. Syphilis itself—particularly in the first and second stages before internal damage might occur—is completely curable.

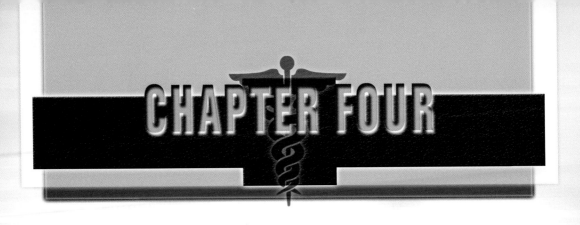

CHAPTER FOUR

Treating Syphilis

When syphilis first began spreading through Europe in the early 1500s, diseases were viewed as poisons that had invaded the body. The three main methods for getting rid of them were bleeding, sweating, and purging (cleansing the body's insides of impurities by taking medicine that provoked vomiting and elimination of such substances).

MERCURY

Bleeding often involved opening up a patient's veins and allowing infected blood to flow into a basin. In some cases, leeches—a type of bloodsucking worm that lives in rivers, lakes, and marshes—were applied to a patient's skin and left to suck out the infected blood. Meanwhile, a common way of provoking sweating and purging was to use the chemical mercury. This silvery-white metallic fluid was named after the Roman messenger god Mercury (in ancient Greece he was called Hermes), who was renowned for his speed and mobility. Mercury plasters, a popular medicine at the time, were used on syphilis patients to sweat impurities out of their systems. In order to provoke spitting and vomiting that would rid them of the disease's poisons, patients often drank mercury compounds. Foul-tasting mercury was an extremely unpleasant treatment, not to mention potentially poisonous. Yet these horrible side effects were preferable to the insanity, paralysis, and death that accompanied the last stages of the worst cases of syphilis.

Although mercury can, in fact, prevent syphilis bacteria from spreading, it neither kills the bacteria nor alleviates the disease's symptoms. For this reason, patients unfortunate enough to develop tertiary syphilis inevitably suffered from the disease's worst complications and very often died. Nonetheless, because it had some benefits, mercury remained the common treatment for syphilis until the early twentieth century.

It wasn't until 1909 that a German physician named Paul Ehrlich invented a more effective treatment for syphilis. However, it contained a small amount of the potentially deadly poison arsenic, which could present serious side effects. Still, in 1910, his formula went on the market as a drug called Salvarsan.

PENICILLIN

Penicillin was the first antibiotic (a substance that can destroy microorganisms that infect humans and animals with diseases) to be discovered and put into widespread use as a cure for infections caused by certain types of bacteria. Derived from a type of mold that grows on bread and fruit, penicillin's useful effects were first observed in 1928 by Scottish biologist Sir Alexander Fleming. However, it was only recognized as a treatment for human beings in 1941, following successful experiments by a group of biologists working at Oxford University in England led by Australia's Sir Howard Walter Florey and Ernst Boris

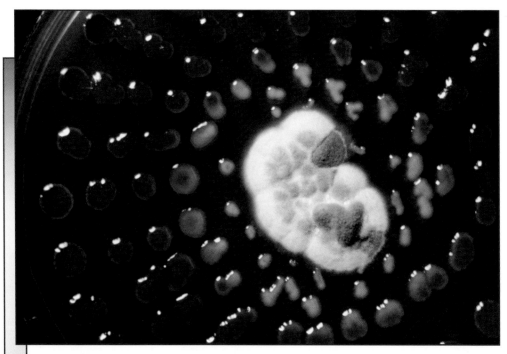

This photograph shows the effect of penicillin (the white substance in the center) on a group of bacteria (shown in red). When applied to a colony of bacteria, penicillin secretes a substance that destroys the bacteria that cause diseases such as syphilis.

Chain of Germany. In 1943, it became a much safer, surefire treatment for syphilis.

By the end of World War II in 1945, penicillin was being manufactured worldwide. For the first time since syphilis was discovered, there was actually a cure. To this day, penicillin remains the most efficient and widely used treatment for the disease.

If identified in the first or second stages (when syphilis has been present in the body for usually less than a year), penicillin is a relatively easy treatment. In the case of primary syphilis, one dose of penicillin is generally all that is required to kill the bacteria. The oldest and most effective method of treatment is to inject the penicillin into each of a patient's buttocks. (Since this can be painful, a painkiller is administered beforehand.) Penicillin can also be taken orally, in pill or capsule form, over a certain time period. This latter method, however, may not be as effective. Not only do some patients not always take the medication according to their doctor's instructions, but some strains of syphilis have recently become resistant to lighter doses of penicillin. For patients with allergies to penicillin (around 10 percent of all people), other antibiotics can be used.

If patients have already experienced the first two stages of syphilis and have had the infection in their bodies for more than a year, subsequent doses of penicillin or other antibiotics taken over a longer period of time (usually about a month) will probably be necessary to kill

The Tuskegee Syphilis Study

In 1932, 399 poor, male, mostly illiterate African American syphilis patients (and 201 uninfected control patients) who lived around the town of Tuskegee, Alabama, were chosen for a study about the disease. A group of scientists and doctors wanted to investigate how syphilis developed over a period of time and how it could be treated. The men who participated in what became known as the Tuskegee Syphilis Study were not informed that they had syphilis or that the disease could be transmitted through sexual activity. Instead, they were told they had "bad blood" and could receive free treatment for their condition.

By the mid-1940s, penicillin had been accepted as a successful cure for syphilis. However, rather than provide antibiotic treatment to the study's subjects, the Tuskegee scientists withheld penicillin and information about it because they wanted to see how syphilis is spread and how it kills. For this reason, when nationwide campaigns to wipe out STDs brought "rapid treatment centers" to Alabama, the Tuskegee scientists prevented the infected men from going to them. Despite warnings from the U.S. Public Health Service to the Centers for Disease Control (CDC) in 1966, this study continued until 1972, when a leak to the press about it shocked and scandalized the nation. By that time, only seventy-four of the test subjects were still alive. Twenty-eight men had died of syphilis and a hundred more had died from syphilis complications. Moreover, forty of the men's wives had been infected and nineteen of their children had been born with syphilis.

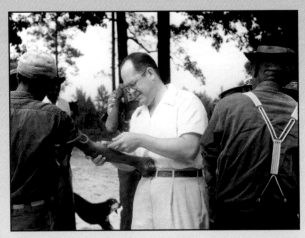

The United States Public Health Service took photographs throughout the forty-two years of the Tuskegee study. All the images have survived, although the names of the participants were never recorded.

Today, the Tuskegee Syphilis Study is viewed as one of the greatest ethical violations of the trust between doctors and patients in a study setting in the United States. As a result, Congress passed specific acts to prevent such horrors from ever happening again.

the bacteria. All antibiotics, including penicillin, are highly controlled drugs that can be prescribed only by a doctor. Neither over-the-counter drugs nor home or natural remedies can cure syphilis. For people with advanced syphilis, who have already begun experiencing more serious internal symptoms, penicillin can kill the syphilis bacteria and prevent further damage. It cannot reverse the effects of damage that has already occurred.

People undergoing treatment for syphilis should have no sexual contact at all until any sores or lesions

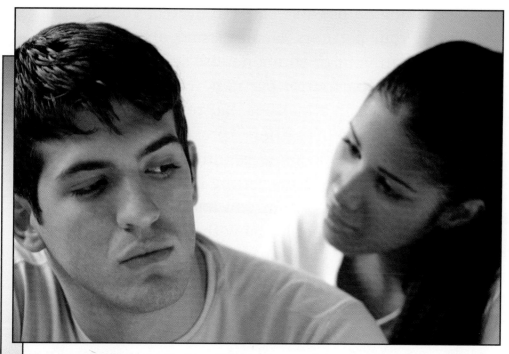

It is often difficult to talk about STDs such as syphilis. However, open and honest communication is essential when people's health and well-being are at stake.

they might have are completely healed. They should also contact any sexual partners they currently have and have had in the past. Although this might be embarrassing or uncomfortable, it is necessary to save people from developing advanced syphilis and from passing it on to others. (Some health departments have partner notification processes and may be able to contact past partners for you. Keep in mind, however, that people who are contacted this way may feel some resentment that they are being told in such an impersonal manner.)

Being sexually active is not just about giving and getting pleasure—it's about being responsible, too. This includes taking all possible steps to protect your health and that of your partners. Health issues are much more important than your or someone else's "reputation." Hopefully, your partner or partners will appreciate your honesty and react in a manner that respects your privacy. Making sure that your partners—present and past—get tested is a sign of respect and is, quite simply, the right thing to do. Even if it means getting in touch with someone you don't like or with whom you had a one-night stand, it is important to let people know they could be at risk. Wouldn't you expect your partner, under similar circumstances, to be honest with you?

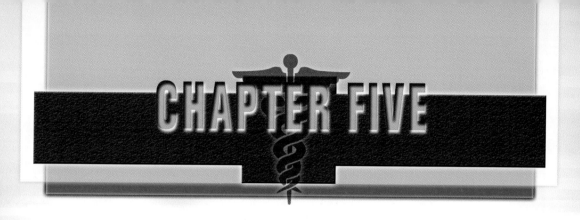

Complications

Although syphilis is easy to diagnose and treat, it is essential that it be detected as early as possible. For this reason, if you even remotely suspect that you or anybody you know could have been exposed to the disease, it is better to be safe than sorry. Getting tested for syphilis will take about an hour out of your life. Aside from saving yourself or someone else from the disease itself, it can prevent the development of some very serious complications that often accompany syphilis if it goes untreated.

CONGENITAL SYPHILIS

Syphilis can be contracted congenitally, meaning an unborn baby can be infected while in a mother's uterus if the syphilis bacteria are in her system. Many times, a pregnant woman might not even know she has syphilis. This is why all women, as soon as they discover they are pregnant, should get tested for syphilis. In fact, when applying for a marriage license in many U.S. states, a

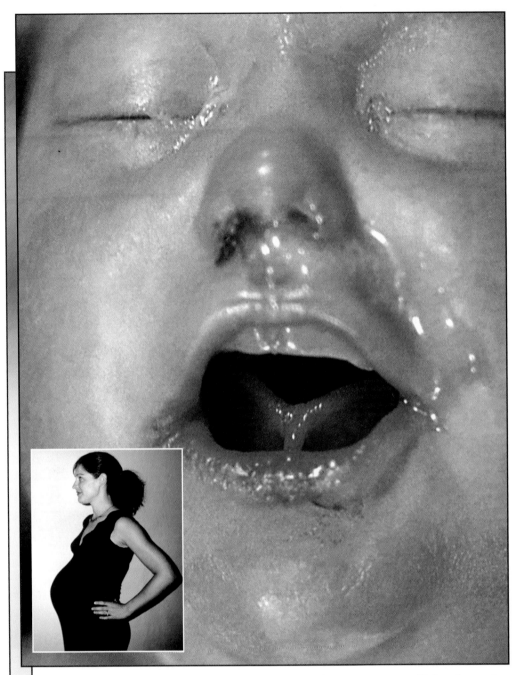

A pregnant woman *(inset)* with syphilis can pass the *Treponema pallidum* bacteria in her system to her unborn baby. The face of the newborn infant pictured shows symptoms of congenital syphilis, including rashes, yellowish skin, and moist, infectious sores.

blood test for syphilis is required as a precaution against spreading the disease to unborn children.

If the test is positive, treatment to kill the bacteria can take place right away. In cases of congenital syphilis, penicillin is considered to be the only antibiotic treatment that is effective. If treated before the sixteenth week of pregnancy, the baby will probably not be affected.

A pregnant woman with syphilis who fails to get tested and treated is taking enormous risks with both her life and that of her baby. Between 25 to 50 percent of pregnant women infected with syphilis suffer miscarriages. Pregnant women with syphilis have about a 40 percent chance of having a stillbirth (a baby that is born dead) or seeing their babies die shortly after birth. Even if a baby whose mother has syphilis is born seemingly healthy, it does not mean that he or she won't suffer from symptoms of syphilis later on. Between 40 and 70 percent of babies whose mothers have syphilis contract the disease. If not treated immediately, the baby can develop severe problems within a period of weeks. Babies with syphilis will often have physical and mental developmental problems, suffer from seizures, experience brain and other internal organ damage, and even die.

MENINGITIS

During the secondary stage of syphilis, it is possible to develop another serious infection called meningitis.

Meningitis affects the meninges, the membranes that cover and protect the brain and spinal cord. In the case of syphilitic meningitis, these membranes are infected by the syphilis bacteria. Syphilitic meningitis is usually a slowly developing, mild to moderate form of meningitis. Its symptoms include a stiff neck, headaches, muscle aches, fever, nausea, and vomiting. In more severe and advanced cases, patients might experience confusion,

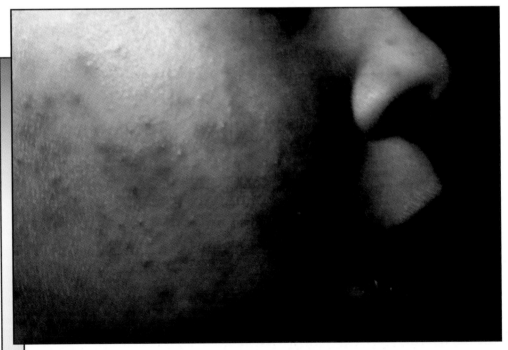

The skin lesions on this young girl's face are a symptom of viral meningitis. Usually, meningitis is caused by bacteria known as meningococcus. However, in the case of syphilis patients, *Treponema pallidum* bacteria can trigger the condition.

irritability, sleepiness, sensitivity to light, blurred vision, and even seizures.

Syphilitic meningitis is treated with penicillin or other antibiotics. With prompt and proper treatment, the infection can be cured and most symptoms will disappear within a short time. However, any serious damage to the nervous system could take weeks or even months to heal.

AIDS AND OTHER STDs

People who have syphilis have a greater chance of becoming infected—and infecting others—with HIV, the human immunodeficiency virus that causes AIDS (acquired immunodeficiency syndrome). In fact, someone with syphilis has two to five times the likelihood of contracting HIV through sexual contact than a healthy person. This is because the HIV virus is transmitted through blood and other body fluids that are released and can be easily exchanged between two people during sex. Because the symptoms of the first two stages of syphilis are chancres and lesions, the skin and mucous membranes that usually serve as protective barriers against infections can bleed easily if touched or rubbed. This makes it much likelier for the HIV virus to be transmitted.

Furthermore, activities that make it possible for someone to contract syphilis, like unprotected sex and needle sharing, are the same activities that make it possible to acquire HIV. If you test positive for syphilis, you should immediately take the precaution of being tested for HIV as well as for other STDs such as gonorrhea and chlamydia. Similarly, if you discover you are HIV positive, it is a good idea to be tested for syphilis.

NEUROSYPHILIS

Syphilis bacteria usually do not affect internal organs until the later tertiary stage of the disease. However, in rare cases if left untreated, people with primary or secondary syphilis might develop a condition called neurosyphilis. It is a disorder of the nervous system that can be quite serious.

Although some people with neurosyphilis may never develop symptoms, others might experience headaches, stiff necks, and fevers that are a result of swelling of the brain's lining. Severe cases of neurosyphilis can lead to seizures, numbness, and vision problems. The best treatment for neurosyphilis is penicillin.

RECURRENCE

Even if you have syphilis and it is treated successfully, there is no guarantee that you will never contract it again. Penicillin and other antibiotics kill the syphilis bacteria. However, if you don't complete your treatment and don't abstain from sexual contact while you still have any open sores or chancres, your syphilis can flare up again. Furthermore, following treatment, if you continue to engage in unprotected sex or other risky behaviors, the chances of acquiring syphilis a second time are just as likely as they were the first time. Even after being successfully treated for syphilis, you, and any partners you might have, should be retested from time to time as a precautionary measure. In general, you should be tested one, two, six, and twelve months after treatment to make sure that the bacteria are truly gone. You should also talk to your doctor about when you can safely have sex again. You don't want to risk infecting your partner and then have him or her give the disease back to you.

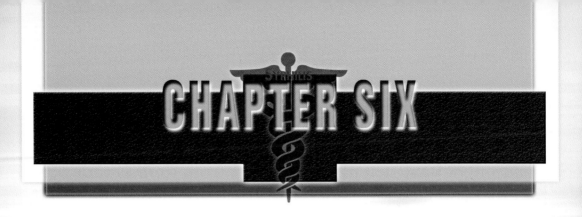

CHAPTER SIX

Prevention

There is no way of avoiding syphilis completely. Even if you don't have sex or share needles, there is a very small possibility of becoming infected. If you kiss someone who has a syphilis chancre on his or her mouth, for example, you could acquire syphilis if the open sore comes into contact with a cut or broken skin. Such cases, however, are extremely rare. The reason syphilis is considered an STD is that it is primarily transmitted through oral, genital, or anal sex.

ABSTINENCE

The best way to protect against any kind of STD is to not have sex. The decision to not be sexually active is called abstinence. Among teenagers, abstinence often gets a bad reputation. Some adolescents think that abstinence is uncool. They think it's a choice made by kids who are afraid of having sex or losers who can't attract a partner. However, such views are far from the truth. Some people might choose not to have sex because of religious, cultural, or personal values. Others simply don't feel they are physically or emotionally ready. Still others might be waiting for a special person or serious relationship before becoming sexually active.

Moreover, choosing abstinence does not mean that you cannot share an intimate and even physical relationship with someone. Hugging, caressing, curling up together, and giving massages are all gratifying and safe ways of expressing your feelings and giving and receiving pleasure.

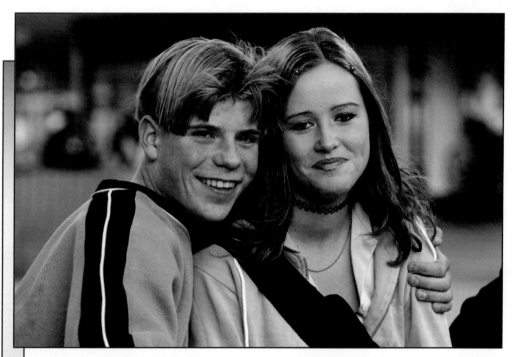

Abstaining from intercourse doesn't mean you can't have a close physical relationship with your partner. In a recent study of urban high school students published by the Sexuality Information and Education Council of the United States (SIECUS), over a third of abstinent adolescents admitted to engaging in some form of intimate physical contact in the past year.

SEX AND THE MEDIA

We are increasingly surrounded by images in magazines, in films, on television programs, and on the Internet of people—especially young people—engaging in sexual activity. However, you have to remember that this is fiction, not reality. These characters are almost never shown putting on condoms, getting STDs, or becoming pregnant, but in real life such things happen all the time. No matter what your friends or other people might say, having sex does not make you an adult. And those who have sex thinking it will make them feel cool or grown-up usually end up feeling disappointed. Making your own individual decision about what is right for you and having the courage to stick to it is the ultimate proof of a mature person.

HAVING SEX

Sex is a big deal. Especially if you're young, and even more so if it's your first time. Your early sexual experiences will affect your entire life. They will help you develop your sexual identity and acquire a degree of comfort with sex that you'll be able to share with future partners. For this reason, you should only have sex if and when you feel absolutely ready.

Deciding Whether or Not to Have Sex

There is no test for deciding when, where, and with whom you should have sex. It is a private and individual

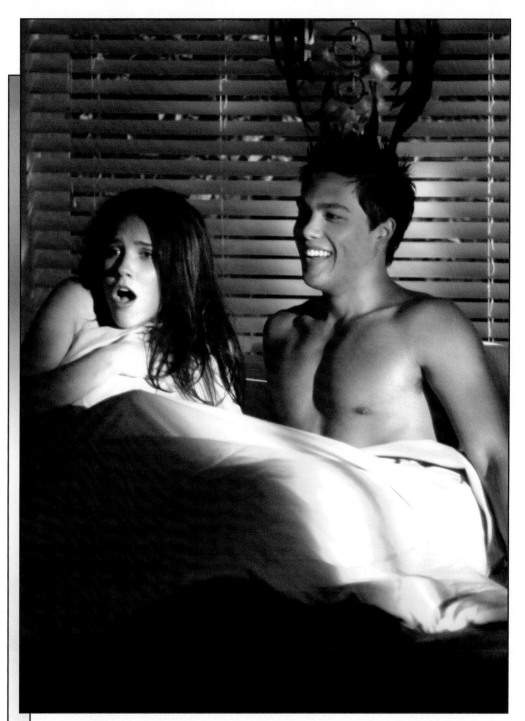

An increasing number of television programs aimed at teenagers address issues of sex and sexuality. Sometimes scenes are quite revealing, such as the one above from the WB's *One Tree Hill*, starring Sophia Bush and Michael Copon.

Some Teenagers Have Sex Because:

- They want to fit in

- It feels good

- It's "cool" to have sex

- It's easier to have sex than to discuss it or say "no"

- They want to feel close to someone

- They feel peer pressure or that everybody's "doing it"

- They're in love

- They're curious and want to experiment

(Source: http://www.iwannaknow.org, operated by the American Social Health Association)

Which of these reasons do you think are good or bad reasons for having sex?

decision that should be discussed openly and honestly with your partner. It should take into account many factors, ranging from how you feel about your partner to how you think you'll feel about yourself afterward. If you're having doubts and feeling confused, try talking to an adult you respect and trust, such as a parent, an older sibling or other relative, a family doctor, or a therapist.

It's important to remember that sex is not a game, a contest, or a competition. It is not something you owe somebody or that you should do in order to be liked.

You should never feel pressured into having sex by your partner or your friends.

Practicing Safer Sex

If and when you decide you want to have sex, you should make sure that you and your partner have discussed and taken all necessary precautions to make the experience pleasurable and safe for both of you. There is no such thing as 100 percent safe sex. There are steps you can and should take, however, to minimize your risk. Safer sex means:

- Limiting your number of partners and knowing their sexual histories (and whether they have been tested for syphilis and other STDs) before starting a sexual relationship.
- Discussing (beforehand) what you are comfortable doing and not doing with your partner.
- Correctly using latex condoms for all types of sex (oral, vaginal, or anal), from beginning to end, every time, along with a proper birth control method (such as an oral contraceptive).
- Never reusing a condom.
- Not having sex while under the influence of drugs and/ or alcohol, since they can alter your perception and cause you to do things you wouldn't usually do.

Contrary to what many people believe, having pro-tected sex does make sex more pleasurable and more

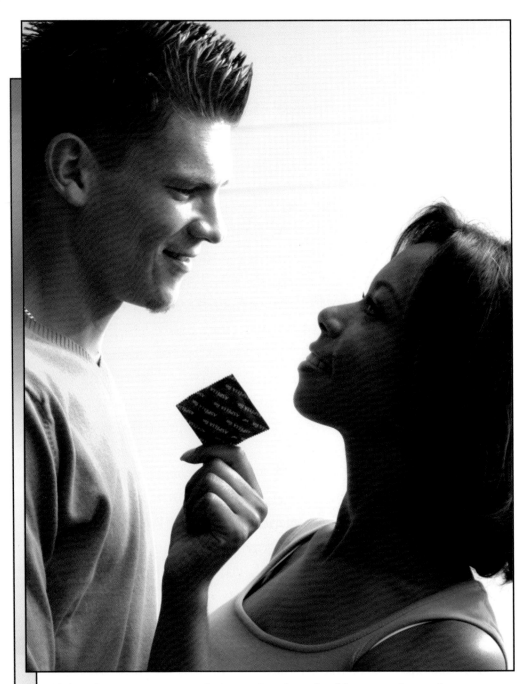

Although many young people know that they should use condoms, they are often embarrassed to buy them, let alone use them. According to a 2004 *People* magazine and NBC poll, only 67 percent of sexually active teens between the ages of thirteen and sixteen said that they use a condom every time they have sex.

relaxing. Not taking precautions will leave you stressed out and nervous during sex because, at the back of your mind, you will know that you are taking a dangerous risk. Condoms don't offer 100 percent protection from syphilis. However, they are the best protection for sexually active people because they provide barriers against the exchange of body fluids.

The frustrating thing about the spread of syphilis and other STDs is that most people know about protecting themselves. However, they often choose not to take precautions out of embarrassment ("I don't want to bring it up"), carelessness ("I forgot condoms"), recklessness ("If it's just this once, nothing will happen"), getting caught up in the heat of the moment, or being under the influence of drugs and/or alcohol. Being aware and responsible is one of the best ways of ensuring that syphilis becomes a disease of the past.

THE FUTURE

Scientists are already investigating many ways to achieve the goal of wiping out syphilis in North America during the twenty-first century. In an effort to reduce the spread of the disease, researchers are working to develop a preventive vaccine, like a flu shot, that would protect people from acquiring syphilis. Also in the works is a diagnostic test that would examine a sample of saliva or urine for the disease. Although home test kits for syphilis exist and are sold over the Internet, their results are not proven to be

Lúcia's Story

Lúcia is a high school student from a strongly religious family. Her dad is from Haiti, her mom is Mexican, and both were raised as strict Catholics. For them, sex before marriage is a sin. However, Lúcia's friends were always talking about sex. Many of them were having sex as well. By the time she was fourteen, Lúcia really was torn. On one hand, she felt guilty about wanting to have sex, but on the other hand, she felt pressure to become a "woman."

Like many of her friends, Lúcia spent a lot of time chatting on the Internet. She posted a profile and a photo on the Web, and engaged in some online flirting. So much talk about sex made her curious, and eventually she decided to meet a guy who seemed interested in her. Alan was older and had his own apartment. The first few times they met, they just kissed and fooled around. However, as weeks passed, things got more intimate. Lúcia came to feel she could trust Alan. They eventually had sex, but they didn't use a condom. Lúcia was worried about becoming pregnant or getting AIDS, but Alan promised that since he didn't ejaculate in her, there was no risk.

Several weeks after they first had sex, Lúcia saw that there was a sore around her crotch. It didn't hurt, but it felt strange. She panicked. She thought God was punishing her and that she had some terrible disease like cancer. She didn't want anyone, including Alan, to know and she stopped wanting to have sex. Of course, Alan got suspicious and Lúcia ended up showing him the sore. He looked worried and advised her to go to a walk-in clinic to have it checked out. He gave her the address of one but said he was too busy to go with her.

Lúcia was nervous at the clinic, but the health workers were very kind. A nurse asked her questions about what she and Alan had done together. When she said they had been having sex, the nurse asked if they used condoms. Lúcia admitted they hadn't, and the nurse said how important it was to always use a condom. After they finished talking, Lúcia had a blood test, which hardly hurt at all.

When Lúcia got home, she called Alan, but he didn't return her call. She tried him several more times, with the same result. She looked for him online, too, but couldn't find him. She didn't understand why he was avoiding her.

A week later, she went back to the clinic, and the nurse told her that she had syphilis. Lúcia was scared because she thought that syphilis was something people died from. She was relieved to hear that after two shots of the antibiotic penicillin, she would be completely cured.

Although Lúcia was glad she was going to be OK, she was angry that Alan had infected her and hurt that he suddenly wasn't speaking to her. She wondered if he even knew he had syphilis. Had he gotten it from someone else while they were together, or had he been infected for a long time? Even though she was upset by the way he had treated her, she didn't want him to continue infecting other people. She sent him an e-mail telling him to get tested.

accurate. Therefore, the government has not officially approved any of these kits.

In terms of treatment, researchers are working toward creating a safe and effective single-dose antibiotic pill or capsule that can cure syphilis. This would please people who hate painful injections as well as those who are allergic to penicillin.

Ultimately, the available medical technology and knowledge about the disease are already advanced enough to eliminate syphilis. With the responsible efforts of today's generation of young people, this dream can certainly become a reality.

GLOSSARY

abstinence The decision not to have any kind of sexual intercourse.

altar A raised structure upon which religious sacrifices can be offered to gods, saints, and other divinities.

antibiotic A medication that destroys microorganisms such as bacteria that infect humans and animals with diseases.

antibodies Proteins in the blood that fight foreign bacteria, viruses, and parasites that attack the body's systems.

cavity A hollow area.

chancre A dull red, hard, open sore.

congenital Relating to a condition that is present at birth through hereditary or environmental factors.

diagnose To identify a disease from its signs and symptoms.

latent Hidden; present but not visible.

latex An emulsion of synthetic rubber used to make condoms.

secrete To generate a substance from cells or bodily fluids.

stillbirth When a baby is born dead.

symptom A sign or indication of disorder or disease.

FOR MORE INFORMATION

Advocates for Youth
2000 M Street NW, Suite 750
Washington, DC 20036
(202) 419-3420
Web site: http://www.advocatesforyouth.org/youth/
     health/stis/types.htm#syphilis
Advocates for Youth creates programs and policies that help
young people make informed and responsible decisions
about their sexual health. Its Web site includes information
about sex, sexuality, and STDs.

American Social Health Association (ASHA)
P.O. Box 13827
Research Triangle Park, NC 27709-3827
(919) 361-8400
(800) 227-8922 (STI Resource Center Hotline)
Web site: http://www.ashastd.org
ASHA is the U.S. authority on information pertaining to
STDs and their consequences. Its Web site includes a
wealth of information on STD transmission, prevention,
testing, and treatment, as well as tips on safer sex and
condom use and links to help groups.

Centers for Disease Control and Prevention (CDC)
Division of STD Prevention (DSTDP)
P.O. Box 6003
Rockville, MD 20849-6003
(800) 232-4636
Web site: http://www.cdc.gov/std/syphilis
The CDC is a government organization whose role is to protect the health and safety of all Americans, provide essential medical services, and control the spread of diseases. The CDC supports research on a variety of infections, including syphilis, the results of which are published on its Web site.

Public Health Agency of Canada
130 Colonnade Road
A.L. 6501H
Ottawa, ON K1A 0K9
Canada
Web site: http://www.phac-aspc.gc.ca/std-mts/
    syphilis_e.html
This national organization works with local governments and health-care providers to improve and maintain the sexual health of Canadians by preventing and controlling STDs. Its Web site is a good source of information featuring recent research and statistics.

HOTLINES

In the United States

National STD/AIDS Hotline: (800) 342-2437
Planned Parenthood Hotline: (877) 4ME-2ASK (463-2275)
    open Monday–Friday, from 9:00 AM–6:00 PM

In Canada

STD/HIV/AIDS Helpline: (800) 668-2437 (Ontario); (866)
    521-7432 (Quebec); (800) 661-4337 (British Columbia)
    Numbers for other provinces and territories can be
    found at http://www.aidssida.cpha.ca/english/
    links_e/index.htm

WEB SITES

Due to the changing nature of Internet links, the Rosen
Publishing Group, Inc., has developed an online list of
Web sites related to the subject of this book. This site is
updated regularly. Please use this link to access the list:

http://www.rosenlinks.com/lsh/syph

FOR FURTHER READING

Bell, Ruth. *Changing Bodies, Changing Lives: A Book for Teens on Sex and Relationships*. 3rd ed. New York, NY: Three Rivers Press, 1998.

Gravelle, Karen. *The Period Book: Everything You Don't Want to Ask (But Need to Know)*. New York, NY: Walker and Company, 1996.

Gravelle, Karen. *What's Going on Down There? Answers to Questions Boys Find Hard to Ask*. New York, NY: Walker and Company, 1998.

Jukes, Mavis. *It's a Girl Thing: How to Stay Healthy, Safe, and in Charge*. New York, NY: Alfred A. Knopf, 1996.

Madaras, Lynda. *What's Happening to My Body? Book for Boys: The Growing-Up Guide for Parents and Sons*. 3rd ed. New York, NY: Newmarket Press, 2001.

Madaras, Lynda. *What's Happening to My Body? Book for Girls: The Growing-Up Guide for Parents and Daughters*. 3rd ed. New York, NY: Newmarket Press, 2000.

Shmaefsky, Brian. *Syphilis* (Deadly Diseases and Epidemics). New York, NY: Chelsea House Publications, 2003.

Westheimer, Ruth. *Dr. Ruth Talks to Kids: Where You Came From, How Your Body Changes, and What Sex Is All About*. New York, NY: Aladdin, 1998.

BIBLIOGRAPHY

Advocates for Youth. "Syphilis." Retrieved November 2005 (http://www.advocatesforyouth.org/youth/health/ stis/types.htm#syphilis).

American Social Health Association. "Syphilis." Retrieved November 2005 (http://www.ashastd.org/sitemap.cfm).

Birnbaum, Nina R., Ronald H. Goldschmidt, and Wendy O. Buffett. "Resolving the Common Clinical Dilemmas of Syphilis." *American Family Physician*. April 15, 1999. Retrieved November 2005 (http://www.aafp.org/afp/ 990415ap/2233.html).

Boockvar, Kenneth. "Syphilis." Retrieved November 2005 (http://www.cpmc.columbia.edu/whichis/private/ aim/21RPR.html).

Centers for Disease Control and Prevention. "Syphilis." Retrieved November 2005 (http://www.cdc.gov/std/ syphilis).

Hecker, Alana. "The History of Syphilis." Retrieved November 2005 (http://homepages.udayton.edu/ ~santamjc/winter99-4/alanahecker.htm).

Kidshealth.org. "Syphilis." Retrieved November 2005 (http:// kidshealth.org/parent/infections/std/syphilis.html).

The Merck Manual of Diagnosis and Therapy. "Syphilis." Retrieved November 2005 (http://www.merck.com/

mrkshared/mmanual/section13/chapter164/
164d.jsp).

PBS Online. "The Lost Children of Rockdale Country."
Retrieved November 2005 (http://www.pbs.org/
wgbh/pages/frontline/shows/georgia).

PBS Online. "The Syphilis Enigma." Retrieved November
2005 (http://www.pbs.org/wnet/secrets/case_
syphilis).

Public Health Agency of Canada. "Syphilis." Retrieved
November 2005 (http://www.phac-aspc.gc.ca/std-mts/
syphilis_e.html).

INDEX

A

abstinence, 46–47
AIDS, 43
antibiotics, 33–37, 44, 55

C

Centers for Disease Control and
    Prevention (CDC), 13, 36
chancres, 22–24, 31, 46
chlamydia, 44
Columbus, Christopher, 14–16, 28
condoms, 51–53, 54
congenital syphilis, 10, 39–41

G

gonorrhea, 44

H

HIV, 43–44

L

latent stage syphilis, 26

M

meningitis, 41–43

N

needle sharing, 9, 43, 46
neurosyphilis, 44

P

primary syphilis, 22–24

S

safe sex, 13, 51–53
secondary syphilis, 24–26
syphilis
    complications from, 39–45
    detection of, 6, 28–31
    diagnosis of, 22–31
    forms of, 10
    infection rates of, 6, 13
    myths and facts about, 10
    names for, 17
    origins of, 14–21
    and pregnancy, 9–10, 39–41
    preventing, 46–55
    recurrence of, 44
    spread of, 7–8, 9, 10, 46
    stages of, 22–28
    symptoms of, 22–28
    treatment of, 32–38

T

tertiary stage syphilis, 26–28
Treponema pallidum, 7, 10
treponemes, 10
Tuskegee Syphilis Study, the, 36

ABOUT THE AUTHOR

Adam Winters was born in Texas and grew up in Canada, where he attended McGill University. As a writer, he has contributed to numerous magazines and newspapers throughout Canada and the United States. He has published various books for Rosen, including several dealing with topics related to teenage sexuality, relationships, and health issues.

PHOTO CREDITS

Cover, p. 4 © www.istockphoto.com/ericsphotography; cover, pp. 1, 4 (silhouette) © www.istockphoto.com/jamesbenet; p. 1 (inset) CDC/Dr. Edwin P. Ewing, Jr.; p. 5 Still Picture Branch, National Archives and Records Administration; pp. 8, 9 © John R. Foster/Photo Researchers, Inc.; p. 11 Centers for Disease Control and Prevention, Sexually Transmitted Disease Surveillance, 2004, Atlanta, GA: U.S. Department of Health and Human Services, September 2005; p. 15 National Museum of Health & Medicine, Armed Forces Institute of Pathology (AFIP 563); p. 16 © Historical Picture Archive/Corbis; p. 19 Bibliothèque Nationale, Paris, France, Giraudon/Bridgeman Art Library; pp. 23, 42 CDC; p. 25 © CNRI/ Photo Researchers, Inc.; p. 27 CDC/Susan Lindsley; p. 29 © LWA-Stephen Welstead/Corbis; p. 34 © Biophoto Associates/Photo Researchers, Inc.; p. 36 National Archives and Records Administration Southeast Region, Records of the Centers for Disease Control and Prevention, RG 442, Tuskegee Syphilis Series; p. 37 © Medioimages/PunchStock; p. 40 CDC/ Dr. Norman Cole; p. 40 (inset) © Charles Gullung/zefa/Corbis; p. 47 © Atlantide Phototravel/Corbis; p. 49 © Warner Bros/courtesy Everett Collection; p. 52 © AJPhoto/Photo Researchers, Inc.; back cover (top to bottom) CDC/Dr. E. Arum, Dr. N. Jacobs, CDC/Dr. Edwin P. Ewing, Jr., CDC/Joe Miller, CDC/Joe Miller, CDC/Dr. Edwin P. Ewing Jr., CDC.

Designer: Nelson Sá; **Editor:** Elizabeth Gavril
Photo Researcher: Jeffrey Wendt